"STUDENT SURGERY MANUAL"

"DEPARTMENT OF SURGERY"

NAME OF INSTITUTION:

STUDENT NAME:

ROLL No.:

ACADEMIC YEARS:

"With Regards & Thanks For 'Study Materials', 'Formats' Consulted And The Moral Support, To Bring It To You'.

COMPILED BY

Prof.(Dr.)Anil K. Sahni

M.S., F.I.C.S., Advanced D.H.A.

SURGEON, UROLOGIST, ENDOSCOPIST,
LITHOTRIPSY SPECIALIST.

Life Member :

Austrian Medical Society

The Association Of Surgeons Of India

Delhi Urological Society

Association Of Minimal Access Surgeons Of India

International Association Of Gastr0-Endosurgeons

Medical Council Of India Reg.No.: 3599(06.01.2005) / 27417(30.05.1983)U.P.

Address: A-1/F-1 Block-A Dilshad Garden
Delhi-110095 India

Mobile : 09873083100

E-Mail : dranil_sahni@yahoo.co.in
dranil_sahni@hotmail.com

"PREFACE"

<u>Comprehensive Update</u>, Comprising Latest Clinico-Investigatory Methodology,
Surgical Pathology,Surgical Radio-Diagnosis,Surgical Instruments, Records Etc.,
With '<u>Additional Chapters</u>': '<u>Paediatrics</u>' & '<u>Female Surgical Patients</u>'.<u>In An Attempt</u>
<u>To Prepare Concise Latest 'Study Material</u>',The Data Available From Various Esteemed
Pioneer Medical Colleges & Teaching Hospitals Publications Etc.,
<u>Have Been Intensively Revised With The Discretion, In Regards To</u> –

- 'Printing Errors'
- The Clinical Approach Methodology
  (Clinical History, Cl. Exam. & Especially The Investigations & Tt.)
- The Necessary Relevant Additions:e.g Recently Available,Very UseFul & Hence Frequently Used
  <u>Radio-Diagnostics</u> (USG, CT, CECT, MRI, Various Different Scans Etc.)& Other Latest <u>Laboratory</u>
  <u>Investigations</u>(Immunology, Serology, Hormonal Assays,Tumor Markers Etc.),
  Including <u>FNACs</u>:With Their <u>Established UseFulness</u> In Regard To Offered Simple, Safe,
  Non/ Minimally Invasive Procedures, With Negligible/Minimal Complications/False Results,
  Specifically Diagnosing The Various Different Disease Processes.
- HowEver,The Classical Methods, Clinical Tests Questionaire, Previously Used ? Obsolete
  Investigations Etc, Have Been Retained,
  To Offer Students An Idea About Senior Examiners.
- The 'Instruction To Students' & Other Topics Have Been Revised,
  Edit Formatted To Facilitate Understanding Of Immediate Needs
  & Learning Ethical Practice & Human Values.
- The Simple, Illustrative Sketch Diagrams Pertaining To,
  Various Body Systems Have Been Added,
  To Facilitate Understanding & Practicing For,

Depicting Different Clinical Disease Manifestations.
<u>The Informative Additional 'Study Material' Chapters,</u>
 Of Important Frequent Need, OtherWise Not Readily Available Include:

      i.<u>Lymthatic System, Lympth Nodes</u> Including Recent
      Cl. Entity Terminologies: <u>Lympthangitis & LympthOedemas,</u>
      With Cl. History, Cl.Exam, Invs Etc. & <u>Illustrative 'Sketch Diagrams'.</u>
      ii.<u>Clinical Approach Methodology</u> For '<u>Paediatric Patients'.</u>
      iii.Clinical Approach Methodology For '<u>Female Surgical Patients'.</u>

The Following <u>Differently Available 'Surgical Exercises'</u> Topics,
A Very Important Necessary Help Especially For Practical Clinical Exams,
Have Been Compiled Together,With <u>Comprehensive 'Study Material Important Notes',</u>
Arranged Systematically To Facilitate Learning Understanding,
In The Beginning Of Exercises For:i.Surgical Pathology ii.Surgical Radio-Diagnosis
      iii.Sugical Instruments With OPD,OT,Special Cases Duty Details
& Log Book. . . O.T (Major,Minor,Local, Regional,General Anaesthesia Etc.) InternShip,
Residency, Speciality Posting Records --- .

Prof.(Dr.)Anil K.Sahni
M.S, F.I.C.S, Advanced D.H.A
Surgeon, Medical Teacher

APPRAISAL FOR
STUDENTS' SURGERY MANUAL

Hide Details **FROM:**Sunil Chumber
TO:dranil_sahni@yahoo.co.in   Message flagged
Monday, 6 August 2012 8:09 AM

Dear Dr Anil Sahni,

Let Me Congratulate You On Your Interest For Improvement Of Education And Skills Of Students.

The Workbook Will Certainly Improve The Performance Of Students In Both Short Term As Well As Long Term.

Have a nice day.

DR SUNIL CHUMBER
AUTHOR-"ESSENTIALS OF SURGERY"
 SURGERY DEPTT.
AIIMS, N.DELHI.

"CONTENTS"

"SURGERY CURRICULUM"

The Clinical Postings Of Students, In The Department Of Surgery Are After Passing First Professional Examination, For Variable Periods In Each Term Or Semester.
During These Postings, Students Are Posted In The **Surgery Wards And Outpatients' Department (OPDs). A Record Of The Cases**, That The Student Has Seen Or Worked-Up During These Posting,Is **Maintained, To Familiarize** The Student To The **Working Of The Department/Unit,**The **Approach To The Patient** And Subsequent **Management**.

The Students Are Advised To **Note Down** The Salient Features Regarding Patients, As In Clinical Case Teachings Or Discussions With The Senior Residents And The Faculty Members.The Logbook, Thus Prepared Will Help The Student To **Maintain Records** And Is **Very Useful**, For **Revisions During Final Examinations**.

'INSTURCTIONS TO STUDENTS'

Following Are The Instructions To Follow During Postings In Department Of Surgery:
Students On Arriving For The **Surgical Postings**, Must Contact The
Senior Resident/Registrar/Faculty Member For
The Beds Allottements & Other Schedules.
They Are Supposed To Be Responsible For Patients Who Are Admitted On These Beds, For The Duration Of Their Postings.
Duties Of Students With Respect To The Patients On **Alloted Beds** Are As Follows:
1.To **Write History** And Perform A **Physical Examination** & Carry Out All **Instructions** Given To Them By Respective Junior And Senior Resident.
2.To Conduct & Or Carry Out **Laboratory Tests** Advised For These Patents.

3.To **Present** These Patients **On The Rounds**.
4.**To Act As Assistant** In Any Surgical Procedure
& Or Operation Upon These Patients.
5.**To Record** The Daily 'Progress Notes' Of The Patient And Treatment Result Outcome.
Students Should Reach Wards **In-Time, After 'Morning Lecture'.**
- To Be Present At The Rounds On 'Teaching Days'.
- On '**Operation Days**', They Should Be Present In The Operation Theatres, To Assist In The Patients Present On Their Beds.
A Student Whose Case Is Scheduled For Operation, Should Report Punctually At 8:30 Am (Or Whatever Time) To Assist In The Operation.
In The **Evenings**, Students Should Complete Their Histories, Physical Examination, Progress Notes, Etc. And Attend The Evening Rounds Or Other Classes As May Be Arranged. They Should Themselves Take The Initiative To Arrange For **Evening Clinics**,
Extra Classes With The Senior Residents And Faculty Members.
All Work In The Wards Must Be **Completed** By 7:00-8:00 Pm, Or **As Schedule**, And Students Should Leave Thereafter Unless Asked To Stay For Any **Specific Duties** By Authorized Persons.

'HISTORY AND PHYSICAL EXAMINATION'

A '**Detailed History**' Of The Present And Past Illness, Family History Etc. Must Be Obtained, As Far As Possible, The Sequence Of Events Should Be Clearly Brought Out.
All The Symptoms, Described By The Patient Should Be Patiently Attended, Irrespective Of The Fact That May Seem To Have No Relation With The 'Probable Diagnosis', Needed Leading Questions Pertaining To Paticular 'Differntial Diagnosis' Are Then Carefully Asked And Noted.

A Complete 'Physical Examination' Should Be Carried Out.

For (P/R)Rectal Examination, Supervision Of Teacher & Or Complete Knowledge About Methodology Etc.Is Recommended.

Tact, Discretion & Utmost Gentleness Is To Be Employed During Examination,
At All Times. Particularly While Dealing Acute, Inflammatory, Painful Conditions & Respecting The Fact That Neoplasms May Be Disseminated By Injudicious Palpation.

Examination Of Operated Patients Need, 'Special Precautions', In Regard To Dressing, Drainage & Other Tubings Etc.

Patients Are Precious **'Study Material Resources'**,In No Circumstances Previlege To Deal Them, Should Be Disgraced Or Subjected To Abuse.Maintaining The **'No Harm Done' Attitude**, In Case Of 'Doubts' Consultation Advices From Teacher & Or Immediately Available Senior Staff , Should Be Seeked.

The Careful History Taking And Physical Examination Recorded, In The Systematic Methodolgy, Is Followed By Consideration Of:
 (1)**Salient Features**
 (2) Impression About The **Clinical Diagnosis And The Differential Diagnosis**
 (3) Suggested **Investigations** Wih Their Purpose,
And
 (4) The **Line Of Treatment** To Be Followed.
    No History Would Be Regarded Complete,
       Unless It Is Noted Down In Writing.

'OPERATION'

Honest Observation Of Basic Norms Of Operation Theatre, To Maintain Asepsis By;
-Changing Clothes,Shoes Etc. As Available & Advised,
-Using Sterile'Caps' & 'Masks',

-Retaining Restriction Entry While Suffering From Upper Respiratory Tract,
 Skin Infection & Or Other Contagious Diseases.
Every Opportunity To **Assist Operation**, Should Be Seeked With Responsible Welcome, As It Provides:
-Training In Surgical Asepsis,Accuaintance
 With Norms & Appliances Etc.
- First Hand Knowledge Of Certain Surgical
 Procedures,
- Most Valuable Experience To Have A Close
 View Of The Pathological Condition And
 Correlate It With The Clinical Findings.

Consultation, Supervision Of A Teacher & Or Immediately Available Senior Staff, Is Strongly Recommended , Before Proceeding With The Patient & Or Sorrounding Appliances Etc.
'PROGRESS REPORT'

Based Upon, Regular Daily Visits To The Patients,
 - **Complete** Knowledge Of The **Progress
  (Vital Parametres Etc.**),
 - Methods Of **Diagnostic Procedures & Treatment**(Conservative,Operative…),
  Blood Transfusion Notes Records,
  As Instituted,
 -**Any Complication** During Pre-Operative & Or
  In Post-Operative Period, Details…
  Are **Closely Observed & Recorded** In The
  History Sheet Of Each Case,Every Day In
  Ordinary Cases And Twice A Day In Serious
  Cases.
Students Are Advised To Approach The Resident For Any Information About Patients.

All **Hospital Records** Of The Patients Are **Confidential** And Should Not Be Communicated,**Special Precautions** Are Needed To Be Observed,
In Cases Involving **DC(Death Certificate), MLR/MLC(Medico-Legal Record Case), PI(Police Information), Autopsy(Post-Mortem) Etc.**

'POSTINGS IN THE OPDs'

During The Posting In The **OPDs Of The Department Of Surgery,**
The Different Semesters Students Must Reach In Time And Go To Various Alloted OPDs Conducted By The Faculty Members And Residents.

They Should **Closely Observe The Working In The OPDs.,**
Take A **Short History** And Perform **Relevant Physical Examination**
And **Record The Cases** Seen Each Day, As Asked By Teachers.

They Should **Read & Have 'Clinical Teaching'** About These Cases.

'RELATIONS WITH PATIENTS'

Learning To Deal With Patients Is An Extremely **Important Part Of Professional Training**, Needing Courtesy, Cheerfulness, And A Personal Interest In The Patient's Welfare As **'Essentials'.**

Students Must At **All Times Maintain A High Standard Of Decorum** In The Wards And Operation Theatres, And Must On No Account Make Noise Or Behave Improperly
Or Discuss Irrelevant Things Loudly.

Circumstances Of Non- Compliance By The Patients,Should Be **Referred To RSO(Resident Surgical Officer),**
Instead Of Pressing The Matter Themselves.

They **Should Not Discuss** With The Patients Or Their Relations Or Friends **Matters Of Diagnosis, Prognosis, Treatment Etc**.
Questions Concerning Such Should Be Referred To The Senior Resident Or Faculty Member.

INSTRUCTIONS FOR HISTORY WRITING
GASTRIC AND DUODENAL DISEASES (SPECIAL FEATURES)

HISTORY :

(1) **Pain**
Nature : Sudden, colicky, continous
Severity
Duration
Time relationship with meals
Situation
Radiation
Hunger pains
Night pain
Relieved or not by taking food or soda
Relieved or not by vomiting
Releived or not by rest dieting

(2) **Appetite**

(3) **Vomiting**

Preceding or following pain
Voluntary or involuntary
Amount
Nature ? Projectile
Affords relief or not to pain
it is controlled by
rest in bed and fluid diet

(4) **Bleeding**

with or without pain
Amount and frequency
Bright red or coffee coloured
Haemetemesis alone
Haemetemesis with melena
melena alone

(5) **Previous Attacks**

Total Duration
Frequency intermissions
Any restriction of diet
Loss of weight
Loss of working hours in past year

(6) **Previous Treatment**

EXAMINATION :

General : Anaemia or cachexia septic focus
Local :
Inspection : Lump
Peristalsis
Palpation : Tenderness
Rigidity
Lump-Consistency
Surface
Edges
Relations
Succussion splash
Size of stomach
Liver
Rest of abdomen
Fluid

Rectal Examination

Lymph nodes

SPECIAL EXAMINATION :
(1) Examination
Hb%
R.B.C. Count
(2) Urine analysis
(3) Fractional Test meal
Position of stomach and Duodenum
Size
Shape
Contour-Outline of rugae
Niche
Notch
Filling defect
Motility, Obstruction

(4) Endoscopy:
Gastro-Duodenoscopy
ERCP/MRCP Stenting Etc.

Barium Study,CECT

GALL BLADDER (DISEASES)

HISTORY :

SPECIAL FEATURES :
(a) Total duration of illness

(b) Any recent change in sympatomatology
(c) History of gall bladder dyspepsia ?
(d) History of biliary colic ?
(e) History of Jaundice Nature

(f) Has the patient a lump ?
Constantly present Intermittent
Increase in size

(g) History of bouts of every with rigor

Previous Attacks

Frequency
Relative severity and duration
Condition between attack

EXAMINATION :

General : Anaemia
Jaundice
Loss of weight
Lymphadenopathy

Abdominal :

Inspection : Lump
liver

Palpation : Lump Liver
Tenderness
Rigidity
Fluid
Any other lump abdomen

Rectal Examination

SPECIAL INVESTIGATION :

(a) **Urine Examination :**
Bile Salts
Bile Pigment
Urobilinogen

(b) **Stool :** Colour

(c) **Blood Examination :**

R.B.C.& Hb%
W.B.C.-Total and Differential
Serum Protein A.G. Ratio
Serum Bilirubin
Icteric Index
Vanden Bergh Test
Serum Alkaline phosphates
Thymol Turbidity

(d) **X-ray Examination :**
Plain X-ray
Oral Cholecystography
Double does cholecystography
Intravenous cholecystography
Barium meal study
USG, CECT, CT Scan Etc.

(e) **Fractional Test Meal :**

SWELLING OF BREAST

HISTORY :

Present Condition

(1) Duration of lump
(2) How discovered
(3) Injury
(4) Lump rate of growth of fluctuation
(5) Pain and relation to menstruction
(6) Discharge from the nipple
Bloody Milky, watery or purulent
(7) With pregnancy
with lactation
Age of last child

(8) Pain in bones

Previous Condition

(1) In the breast

(2) Pregnancies if any
Breast fed or bottle fed children

(3) Any previous treatment

PHYSICAL EXAMINATION :

General :

Local-inspection :

Is there a lump visible
Side
Quadrant
Any displacement of breast
Retraction of nipple
Any skin changes- Puckering
Oedema
Ulceration
Nodules

Discharge from nipple

Character
from which quadrant
Any lump visible in axilla or supra
Clavicular fossa
Oedema of the arm
Any Changes in the nipple

Palpation :

Is there a lump palpable with flat of hand
Single or multiple
Is it nodular breast
(a) Tumour : Situation
Size
Consistency
Surface
Edge
Relations-Skin
Pectoral muscles
Chest wall
(b) Characters of ulcerated tumour
(c) Dissemination :
(1) Continuity - Overlying skin
Pectoral muscles
Chest wall
Bones
Parietal Pleura

(2) Lymph nodes both sides
Axillary
Supraclavicular
Mediastinal
(d) Is opposite breast normal ?
(e) Abdomen-Liver enlargement ?

Investigations : FNAC, Mammography. USG Etc.

X-ray : Secondaries
(1) Lungs
(2) Bones specially vertabrate
Pelvis
Long bones

Stage : (1) Clinical preoperative
(2) Post-operative

Therapy : Details of D. X. T. Per or
Post-operative

> Breast Conservation Therapy(BCT):
> Breast Conservation Surgery(BCS): Adjuvant /
> Neo-Adjuvant Chemo-Endocrinal,
> Radiotherapy Regimes

THYROID SWELLINGS

HISTORY

I. Time of onset
Total duration
Relationship with puberty
Rate growth
Pain ?
Any change in size of swelling ?
Is change in size related to menstruation
Any recent change in swelling ?

II. Evidence of pressure symptoms
(a) Dysphagia
(b) Dysarthria
(c) Dysphonia
(d) Dyspohea particularly
nocturnal

III. Evidence of excessive Thyroid activity
(a) Fatigueability
(b) Increased appetite
(c) Irritability
(d) Nervousness
(e) Tremors
(f) Loss of weight
(g) Palpitation
(h) Excessive perspiration
(i) Irregularity in menstrual cycle
(j) Gastrointetinal disturbances
(k) Protrusion of eye ball

(l) Any thyroid crisis
(m) Liking for cold or hot wheather

IV. Evidence of hypoactivity of thyroid :
(a) Increase in weight inspite of poor appetite
(b) Swelling of face and eye lids
(c) Coarse skin
(d) Falling of hair
(e) Mental dullness
(f) Constipation
(g) Irregularity in menstrual cycle

V. General Constitutional symptoms
Loss of weight
Loss of appetite
Weakness
Secondary deposit-Pain
Swelling

VI. Effects of drug therapy and rest in bed
on the swelling and symptoms

Physical Examination :

1. LOCAL (A) Inspection
Swelling in thyroid region
Movement on deglutition
Localized swelling or diffuse
enlargement of thyroid
Smooth uniform unlargement or

irregular
Change in overlying skin
Can you see the lower border of
swelling particularly on deglutition ?
Or does it appear restrosternal ?
Any obvious pulsation ?
Any other swelling in neck ?
Does it move on protrusion of tongue ?

(B) Palpation :

Diffused or localised
Consistency ?
Surface
Edges
Thrill
Can you feel lower border ?
Or is it restrosternal ?
Mobility ? Is swelling fixed to
Deeper structures
Any fixity to skin or sternomastoid
Feel the carotid vessels
Pushed laterally (Benignlesions)
Inability to feel pulsations at the level of
goitre (Maligancy)
Feel trachea
Is it central ?
Or compressed ?
Any enlargement of regional
lymph nodes
character of these lymph-nodes

Percussion : over manubrium sterni ?
Dullness (Restrosternal goitre)

Ausculation :

Bruit over thyroid swelling ?
Evidence of hyperactivity
Wasting ?
Appearance ? Excitable, Nervous
or Irritable.
Termors in Fingers and tongue
Pulse ? Tachycardia
Sleeping pulse rate
Irregularity ?
Temperature
Blood Pressure ?

Eye Signs :

Exophthalmos
Lid retraction (Steel wag's (sign)
Lid Jag (Von Graefe's sign)
Convergence of eye balls (Moebius sign)
Wrinkling of forehead (Joffory's sign)
Examine heart for any cardiac irregularities

Investigations :

(a) Sleeping Pulse rate
(b) A. P. and Lateral X-ray of neck
 Position of trachea
 Any calciication
(c) X-ray of superior mediastinum
 A.P. and lateral
 restrosternal goitre
(d) Laryngoscopy
 Paralysis recurrent larygeal nerve
(e) B. M. R.
(f) Blood cholesterol
(g) Urine analysis
(h) Effect of rest in bed and antithyroid
 drugs.
FNAC, USG Neck, CT Scan Neck, Thyroid Scan Etc.

ANO- RECTAL CASES (SPECIAL FEATURES)

History

Present condition

Duration

Pain

Relation to defaecation

Severity

Duration

Discharge

Character- mucous

 blood-bright or dark

(e) Dysuria

(f) Haematuria
   painless or painful
   Bright Red or altered
   Mixed with urine or apart
   Relationship with micturition
   Shape of clots if any

(g) pyuria

(h) Oliguria

(i) Polyuria

(3) Associated Symptoms :

(a) Fever -
   without or with rigors
   continuous or intermittent

(b) Any other Tubercular focus

(c) Associated disease of Epididymis

(d) Evidence of metastic deposit

(e) Symptoms of uraemia

Physical   Examination :
General :   Does patient look ill,
            anaemic emaciated,
            dehydrated, uraemic

Local :

Abdomen :   Examine upper and
                lower for evidence of
                masses or tenderness

Back :   Costovertebral angle : look
             for masses or tenderness

Male Genitals :

Palpate urethra
Epididymis
Testis
Vas

Prostate
Seminal Vesicles
Base of bladder
Vaginal Examination (Female)
   Urethra
   Base of Bladder

Bimanual Examination of Bladder
   Sometimes the stone is palpable
   Growth of base of bladder and
   its extra vesical extension

Rectal Examination :

Special Examination :

(1) **Blood :** Serial 1, 2, 3, 4, 5, 6
   Urea
   N. P. N.
   E. S. R.
   S. Acid Phosphatase, Prostate Specific antigen (PSA):
                        Free, Total, Ratio

(2) **Urine :**
   Output
   Physical Character
   Urine analysis
   Culture
   Special culture T.B (AFB)
   Guinea-pig-inoculation

(3) **Renal Function Test :**
   Urea concentration
   Urea clearance, Free Total

(4) **Skiagraphy :**
   Straight
   I. V. P.
   Retrograde Pylography
   Cystogram
   Urethrogram
   USG Whole Abdomen (Full Bladder) &
   Post Micturition, Post Void Residue (PVR)
   CECT Abdomen,
   Whole Body Scan, Bone Scan Etc.

(5) **FNAC, Prostate Biopsy: Trucut Etc.**
(6) **Cysto-Uretheroscopy & Proceed.**
(7) **X-ray Chest**
(8) **Tuberculin Test**
(9) **Serology For T.B**
   Elisa For T.B

Mixed with stools or not
Character to stool
Constipation
Diarrhoea
Alternating constipation and diarrhoea
Anything comming down
With or apart from defaecation
Any abdominal condition associated

Previous History :

Previous attacks
Extending over what period

PHYSICAL EXAMINATION

Local Inspection :
Prolapsed piles
Prolapse
Evidence of Pruritus
Sinuses-Discharging
Fissure

Palpation :
No Probe allowed
Condition of external sphincter
Painful, patulous anus or spasm
Thrombosed Haemorrhoids
Internal Opening of fistula
Fissure
Induration external- (between the finger
in the rectum and thumb externally)
Prostate
Mass
Consistency

Surface
Edges
Base
Relations
Ulcer - Surface
        Edges
        Base
        Discharge
Stricture :
Situation
Linar or annular
Size
Consistency
Pouch of Douglas

ABDOMINAL EXAMINATION

Secondary deposits
Evidence of acute or chronic or chronic
intestinal obstruction

SPECIAL INVESTIGATION

i.   Probing
ii. Contrast Radiology : Fistulography
iii. Colour Radiology
iv. Endoscopy   Colonoscopy
              Proctoscopy
              Sigmoidoscopy
v.   Barium Study
     (a) Barium Enema
     (b) After evacuation
     (c) Double contrast media study
vi. In maligancy
     (a) Blood Urea and Nonprotein
         Nitrogen, Tumor Markers Etc.
     (b) I.V.P
     (c) CECT Whole (Upper & or Lower)
         Abdomen, MRI, Other Scans Etc.

GENITO - URINARY CASE (SPECIAL FEATURES)

History

Present Condition

Presenting complaints. Duration.
Onset and Course

(1) PAIN : Relation to micturition
     When - before, during or
            after micturition
     Mode of onset-sudden
                or gradual
     Mode of Termination
     Sudden or gradual

Colicky or continuous
Aggravated by exercise
or not

(2)   URINATION
      (a) Difficulty
      (b) Frequency :   Increased or not
                         Day or night
                         Rest or
                         Exercise
      (c) Dribbling
      (d) Retention :   Acute
         AFB Culture Sputum,Body Fluids   Chronic

(e) Dysuria

(f) Haematuria
painless or painful
Bright Red or altered
Mixed with urine or apart
Relationship with micturition
Shape of clots if any

(g) pyuria

(h) Oliguria

(i) Polyuria

(3) Associated Symptoms :

(a) Fever -
without or with rigors
continuous or intermittent

(b) Any other Tubercular focus

(c) Associated disease of Epididymis

(d) Evidence of metastic deposit

(e) Symptoms of uraemia

Physical Examination :
General : Does patient look ill,
anaemic emaciated,
dehydrated, uraemic

Local :

Abdomen : Examine upper and
lower for evidence of
masses or tenderness

Back : Costovertebral angle : look
for masses or tenderness

Male Genitals :

Palpate urethra
Epididymis
Testis
Vas

Prostate
Seminal Vesicles
Base of bladder
Vaginal Examination (Female)
Urethra
Base of Bladder

Bimanual Examination of Bladder
Sometimes the stone is palpable
Growth of base of bladder and
its extra vesical extension

Rectal Examination :

Special Examination :

(1) **Blood** : Serial 1, 2, 3, 4, 5, 6
Urea
N. P. N.
E. S. R.
S. Acid Phosphatase, Prostate Specific antigen (PSA):
Free, Total, Ratio

(2) **Urine :**
Output
Physical Character
Urine analysis
Culture
Special culture T.B (AFB)
Guinea-pig-inoculation

(3) **Renal Function Test :**
Urea concentration
Urea clearance, Free Total

(4) **Skiagraphy :**
Straight
I. V. P.
Retrograde Pylography
Cystogram
Urethrogram
USG Whole Abdomen (Full Bladder) &
Post Micturition, Post Void Residue (PVR)
CECT Abdomen,
Whole Body Scan, Bone Scan Etc.

(5) **FNAC, Prostate Biopsy: Trucut Etc.**
(6) **Cysto-Uretheroscopy & Proceed.**
(7) **X-ray Chest**
(8) **Tuberculin Test**
(9) **Serology For T.B**
Elisa For T.B

PERIPHERAL VASCULAR DISEASE

History :

(1) Onset- gradual or sudden
(2) Duration
(3) Pain
Present or absent
Change due to posture-elevation
or depression
Change due to external temperature-cold-
warmth
Rest pain
Intermittent Claudications
Muscles involved
How much can he walk ?
It is continuous pain or intermittent
Changes in colour of skin
    Due to posture
Due to external temperature changes
(4) Any history of recurrent minor
infections in fingers and toes ?
(5) An ulceration, gangrene
(6) Wasting of extermity
(7) Evidence of fleeting thrombo phlebitis
(8) Is patient a diabetic
Polyphagia
Polyurea
Polydypsea
(9) Any previous attack in the
(10) Does he smoke ? Since When ?
How much ?
(11) Is he used to any sedatives ?

Physical Examination :
General
Local

Inspection :

(i) Colour of skin
Pallor
Cyanosis
Dusky Colour
Changes in colour due to elevation
despression of limb
(ii) Varicose Veins
(iii) Wasting of limb
(iv) Hairs loss
(v) Conditions of nails
(vi) Ulceration ? Gangrene ?

Palpation :

(1) Skin temperature
any sudden gradient in skin temperature?
(2) Skin nodules or thickening
(scleroderma)
(3) Palpation of main vessels :

Right	Left
Femoral	
Popliteal	
Posterior tibial	
Dorsalis pedis	
Brachial	
Axillary	
Radial	
Ulnar	

Examination of Heart

Special Investigations
(1) Result of elevation of limb
(2) Walking test ? Claudication distance
(3) X-ray of limb - (straight-X-ray)
Calcification of blood vessels
(4) oscillometry
(5) Angiography
(6) Skin temperature studies
(7) Results of paravertebral sympathetic
block or spinal anaesthesia
(8) **Color Doppler's Study**

> Vascular Narrowing,
> Obstruction,? Cause,
> Blood Flow Velocity Etc.

'LYMPHATIC SYSTEM'
Lympth Nodes & Lymphatics

History :

(1) **Onset**

(2) **Duration**

(3) **In cases of Generalized Involvement**
First Affected Group,
Otherwise Involvement of Other Groups.

(4) **Associated Features:** Infection.
Inflammation, Toxicaemia:
Pain, Fever (? Pattern) Etc.

(5) Loss of Weight & Appetite,
Evening Rise Temp.,
Chest Infections,
& other Involved organ Symptoms
for T.B other Infections, Malignancy Etc.

(6) **Primary Focus :**
Associated History : Bacterial : T.B,
Suggestive of Infections Actinomycosis
Sarcoidosis, Brucellosis,
Protozoan: Toxoplasmosis,
Viral : Infection Mononucleosis, HIV Etc.,
Neoplastic: Primary; Lymphoma,
Secondary; Squamous Cell Ca,

Known Primary, Occult Prim.

(7) **Pressure Effects :** Dysphagia,
Swelling, Oedema, Dysnoea,

(8) **Family & Social History of Causative**
& or Associated Diseases.

(9) **History suggestive of :**
(A) Cong. Malformations
(Primary Lymphoedema)
(B) Accuired Obstruction
(Secondry Lymphoedema),
H/O Infections eg Filariasis,
Endemic Elephantiasis
(Podoconiosis) Etc.
Previous Surgery, Trauma Etc.
In the Adjoining Body Regions,
Systemic Cardiovascular Dis.,
Diabetes,Deep Vein
Thrombosis
(DVT),Superficial Vein
Thrombosis (SVT) Etc.

(C) Ac. Sub. Ac., & Chr.
Lymphanigitis

Clinical Exam. : General

Systemic : Esp. Abdomen, Thorax
For Hepato-Splenomegaly,
& Cl. Evident L.N Masses.

Local
Inspection :
Swelling
Overlying Skin
Pressure Effects & or
Lesions
in Adjoining; Drainage Areas

Palpation :
Temp. Tenderness.
No. Site, Size, Shape, Surface,
Consistency, Discrete Or Matted,
Fixity to Overlying skin &
NearBy Structures.Openings,
Discharge Etc.

Investigations :

FNAC

Needle Aspiration for C&S,

Cytology Esp. Maligants Cells.

Peripheral Blood Smear/Film

X-ray Chest PA view

USG Whole Abdomen

CT/CECT Abdomen / Thorax, MRI

Specific Investigations:
-For T.B, HIV & Other Infections
?Maliganancy : Primary, Secondary, ? Occult.

-Biopsy : Excisional, Incisional,
Trucut organ Etc.

-Lymphangiography,

-Isotope Lymopho Scintigraphy Etc.

-Exploratory Laprotomy,
Staging Laprotomy Etc.

'Diagrammatic Illustrations Of Various L.Node Groups With Drainage Areas'

(A) Cervical Lymph Nodes

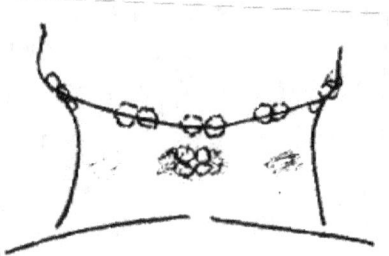

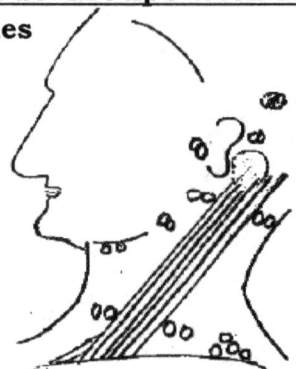

Drainage Area : Scalp, Head, Ear, Nose, Throat, Face, Neck

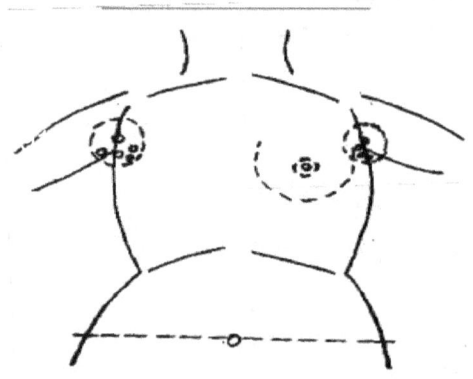

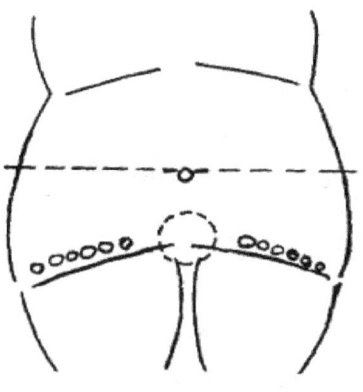

(B) Axillary Lymph Nodes

(C) Inguinal Lymph Nodes

Drainage Area : Ipsilateral Sup. Extremity, Trunk (Ant. & Post. From Clavicle to Umblicus)

Drainage Area : Inf. Extremity, Skin upto Umblicus (Ant. & Post.), Ext. Genitalia, Perineum, Terminal Part Anal Canal, Vagina

(D) Mediastinal, Retro-Peritoneal, Para-Aortic, Mesenteric Etc. Group of L. Nodes

NEUROLOGICAL HISTORY

HISTORY OF PRESENT ILLNESS :

Special features :

Headache

Vomiting

Paresis

Convulsions

Sensory changes

Decreased vision

Urinary disturbances

Defaecation disturbances

GENERAL OBSERVATIONS :

— Position of body, Extremities, head,
— Nutrition
   State of consciousness
Skin : Fine or coarse
   Pigmentation
— HEAD — Inspection — Shape
                    — Veins
   — Palpation — Exostosis
   — Percussion — Tenderness
              — Resonance
   — Auscultation Bruit
   — NECK — Stiffness,

INTELLECTUAL & MENTAL FUNCTION

1. Appearance and Behaviour
2. Emotional state
3. Orientation in place and time
4. Memory
5. General Intelligence

SPEECH :

CRANIAL NURVES :

First Nerve.
1. Subjective — Impairment of smell :
                olfactory hallucinations.
   Objective — Response of each nostril to oil
                of clove.
   2nd nerve
2. Subjective — Impairment of vision generally
                or by field Visual hallucina-
                tions.
   Objective — Acuity of vision
              — Visual field
              — Colour Blindness
              — Endoscopy
3. Subjective : Diplopia
   Objective : External ocular move-
                ments
4. Nystagmus
5. Ptosis
   3rd nerve
       Pupils — Size, equality.
                regularity, Reaction to
                L & A.
   3 — P t o s i s , D i v e r g e n t
   Strabismus
   Diplopia
   Loss of L & A relfex
   4th nerve
   4 — Diplopia on looking down and out
   5th Nerve
   6 — Convergent Strabismus

For these 3 nerves test : 3,4, 6th Nerve

   (a) Movement of eye ball

   (b) Presence of squint

   (c) Presence of diplopia

6   Subjective : Sensation Neuralagia

         Numbness

         Paresthesia

Objective : Sensory-Test facial sensations,
              Corneal
              reflex

   Motor-Deviation of Jaw

      Muscles of mastication

7   Subjective : Facial asymmetry

      Facial spasms

      Loss of taste sensation

      Anterior 2/3 tongue

      Hyperacusis

      Escape of saliva from angle

      of mouth

Objective Motor-Facial Expression
            Wrinkle forehead
            Eye closure
            Showing the teeth

Sensory-Taste sensation
    anterior 2/3 tongue

8. *Cochlear :*

    Subjective : Hearing impairment
          ringing.

    Objective : Tick of watch. tuning
               fork
        Rinne's Test
        Waber's Test
        Otoscopic Examination

VESTIBULAR :

    Subjective : Ataxia, Vertigo, Nausea

    Objective : Nystagmus, swaying.

9. Subjection : Dysphagia

    Objective : Gag reflex-Tickle post
              1/3 Tongue

10. Subjective : Disturbance in swallow-
          ing and speaking
          projectile vomiting

    Objective : Deviation of soft palate
          Laryngeal Paralysis
          Inability to swallow.

11. Cannot shrug shoulder

12. Deviation of protruded tongue
       affected side.
    Not-fibrillations, atrophy

LOCALIZATION CEREBRUM :

FRONTAL – Defective cerebration
          Lack of concentration
          Euphoria
          Personality change
          Insomnia
          Incontinence

Motor Area : Convulsions
          Paresis of paralysis
          Aphasia

Pre-motor : Forced grasping
          Clumsiness

Parietal : Sensation intact or not
          Can he tell shape of
          things?

Occipital : Visual hallucinations

Quadrantic field defect

Temporal – Auditory or visual halluci-
nation

Dream states

Hamianopia

Sensory aphasia

CEREBELLUM LOCALIZATION

Tone of muscles

Speech : Dysarthria present in cerebellar
lesions

? Ataxia) Finger to nose tests

? Asynoigy) Heal to knee

Adiadokokinesis

Romberg's sign

SPINAL CORD

Subjective : Muscle weakness
Walking
Bladder Functions
Rectal Function
sensations
Pain
Sweating

Objective : Upper limb Lower limb

(a) Motor Power
Tone
Nutrition

(b) Attitude

(c) Sensation
Touch
Heat and cold
Pain
Position sense
Vibration sense

(d) Jerks

Superficial – Corneal

Abdominal

Cremasteric

Deep – Knee
Ankle
Biceps
Triceps

Babinski response

Clonus – Ankle
Knee

SPECIAL INVESTINGATIONS

(a) Blood – W. R. and Khan Test

(b) Lumbar Puncture – Pressure –
manometry

Character of fluid

Analysis of C.S.F.

Culture

Special Test on
C.S.F.

(c) Skiagraphic :

(1) Plain X-ray of skull & spine

(2) Cerebral arteriography

(3) Pneumo-Encephalography

(4) Myelography

(5) - CT Scan, MRI & Others
- Muscle Power &
Nerve Conduction Studies Etc.

HEAD INJURIES

History :

Time of Occurence
Loss of Consciousness
Was it immediate ?

_____

Nature of injury :
Cause :

How long did it remain?

Did he become unconscious after regaining consciousness ? It so

Any Wound ?

Any swelling ?

Any haemorrhage from Ear, Nose Mouth ?

Any clear fluid discharge from Ear, Nose or mouth (C.S.F.) ?

Any vomiting ?

Did vomitus cantain blood ?

Any fever ?

Any twitching or Convulsions ?

If so describe in details

Any paralysis

C H A R T S

Any other injury ?

What is the present level of the consciousness
Is he comatose ? (No response) or
response to command - response to
Painful Stimuli

Physical Examination :

Physical examination of an unconscious
patient is always unsatisfactory. Detailed
neurological examination cannot be done.

Time of Admission :

Sign of shock :

Respiration : rapid and shallow, slow
laboured and stertuous
Cheyne Stroke's respiration.

(a) Half hourly Pulse													
(b) 2 hourly B. P.													
(c) 2 hourly temp.													

Pupils : On admission?
- See the size and reaction
  to light in both pupils
  Record changes every 1/2 hour.
- Level of consciousness
  Record change of level of consciousness
  (Very significant if associated with any
  focal signs e.g.
  unilateral pupillary reaction, Hemiplegia)
- Neurological Examination
  Facial asymmetry
  Paralaysis of Extremities ?
  Sphincter Control ?
- Reflexes Knee
  Ankle
  Abdominal
  Plantar response

- Any changes in neurological signs ?
Examine for Presence of Any Injury
Fracture of extremity bones ?
Spinal Injuries ? Chest & Or Abdominal Injuries, Other Injuries
Local Examination :
(a) Swelling ? Haematoma
     Give its characters, Is it pulsatile ?
(b) Wound ? Describe
     Any fracture seen ?
     Any haemmorhage ?
     Any flow of C.S.F.
     Any protrusion of brain matter.
(c) Any fracture ?depressed
(d) Any extravasation of blood in soft tissues
     seen or felt ?
     Black eye ?

Subconjunctival haemmorhage ?
In Neck ?
In Temporalis muscle ?
(Significant in middle meningeal
haemmorhage)

After Recovery From Unconsciousness
    Do a detailed neurological examination
Investigation :
I. X-ray of skull ?
II. Lumbar-Puncture
III. CT Scan Head, MRI & Others

ABDOMINAL EMERGENCIES

History :
Pain : Onset — Any warning
           Time of onset
           Situation
           Radiation
           Nature
           Severity
  What relieves it ?
  Change of situation
  Change of Character

Vomitting :   Type
              frequency
              Quantity
              Quality

Bowels : Absoulte constipation
        Constipation or diarrhoea
        Discharge mucus or blood
        Increased peristalsis
        Visible
        Audible
Has the patient noticed any lump
      recent change

Micturition - Any relation with pain
Has menstruation any relation with pain

Is the patient aware of any hernia ?
    Any recent change in it

History of previous attacks if any

PHYSICAL EXAMINATION

GENERAL
    Facies
    signs of dehydration
    signs of internal haemorhge
    Pulse
    B. P.

Local : Inspection :
    Hernial sites
    Distension situation
        Degree
Evidence of increased
        Peritstalsis
Situation
Diroction

Palpation :

Tenderness
Rigidity
Lump :   Situation
           Consistency
           Surface
           Edges
           Relations
           Mobility

Percussion : Free Fluid
    Free gas (Liver dullness)
    Resonance
    Rolation of gut to the mass

Auscultation :
    Peristalsis
    Pregnancy
    Aneurysm

Pelvic Examination :
    P V
    Rectal Examination

Special Examination :
  (1) Blood Count
  (2) Two enemas - If Indicated
  (3) Straight X-ray of abdomen,
        Erect With Both Domes Diphargm
  (4) Screening Liver abscess
        Subphrenic abscess
  (5) USG Whole Abd.
        (Full Bladder)
  (6) CT/CECT Whole Abd.

CHEST CASE

History :
- (a) Cough
- (b) Fever
- (c) Pain
- (d) Haemoptysis
- (e) Dyspnoea Orthopnea
- (f) Sputum : Amount
  - Character
  - Smell
- Personal or family History of Tuberculosis

EXAMINATION :

1. **General Examination :**
   Anaemia
   Cachexia

2. **Chest Examination**

   Inspection : Shape
   - Bulging
   - Shrinking
   - Movement of chest wall
   - Any restriction local
   - or general

   Palpation : Position of apex beat
   - Position of Trachea
   - Vocal fremitus

Percussion :

Ausculation :

   Character of sound
   Adventitious sounds
   Vocal resonance

INVESTIGATIONS :
(1) **Blood :** Routine blood picture
   E.S.R. Serology : Elisa For T.B, Immunoglobulin Studies,
   Polymerase Chain Reaction (PCR) & Others

(2) **Sputum Examination**
   (a) For A.F.B. (repeated examination)
   (1)
   (2)
   (3)
   (b) Organism
      Culture
   Antibiotic sensitivity

(3) **X-Ray Examination**
   (a) screening
   (b) Radiography : P.A.- and
                     Lateral Films
   (c) Tomography
   (d) Bronchography

(4) **CT Scan Thorax**
(5) **Bronchoscopy :**
(6) **Exercise Tolerance Test**
(7) **Vital Capacity**

FRACTURES : (COMPLETE THE MEDICOLEGAL ASPECTS OF EVERY CASE)

Present Condition :
- Duration
- Cause - Direct Violence
         Indirect violence
         Nature
         Severity

Audible crack
Pain
Loss of Function
Deformity
Ecchymosis
Abnormal mobility

Previous History :
- Other fractures
- Any disease when you suspect
- Pathological fracture

Physical Examination :
(1) **General:** Shock
              Signs of heamorrhage
              Any other visceral or
              bony injury
(2) **Local :** Compare with healthy side
   Inspection : Swelling
                    Deformity

(3)   Biopsy regional lymph Node
(4)   X-Rays :
        Straight A.P. and Lateral Views
        CT Scan, MRI & Others

        Sinogram
        X-Ray Chest
(5)   Biopsy :- Synovial or Bone.

DISEASES OF JOINTS

History :

Present Condition :
  Duration
  Cause to which attributed
  Pain- Sudden or gradual onset
  Severity
  Character-aching
        Night start
  Day or night
  Relation to exercise
  Rigor
  Fever
  Lacking
  Swelling
  Power of limb

Previous History- Inless typhoid
        gonorrhoea
        Attacks as above
        Condition in between
        attacks

Physical Examination :
General : Sepsis - Tonsils, Teeth, Urethra
        Signs of tuberculosis
        syphilis

Local: Inspection
        Limp or peculiarties of gait
        Position of joint
        Deformity

Swelling :   Obliteration of joint
                out-line
Redness of skin
Engorged veins
Wasting of muscles - above the below
Extent of voluntary movements
Abnormal movements

Palpation : Heart
        Tender spot
        Irregulants of Joint out-line
        Fluid
        Creaking

Extent normal movements
  Presence of abonormal movements
  Enlargements of bursae round joint
  Enlargement of lymph nodes
  Measurements

Special Examination:
  X-ray of joints A.P. & Lateral views
        (Both sides)
  X-ray chest
  Blood-Test & Differential W.B.C.
  E.S.R. W.R. & kahn Test
  Specific Serology & Or Immunology
  Tuberculin test, Elisa for T.B. & Others
  Biopsy regional lymph nodes

Aspiration of joint fluid and examination
Synovial Biopsy

'PAEDIATRIC SURGICAL PATIENTS'

Presence of Responsible aware Attendant preferably parents,

Is an important Pre-requisite.

(1) **History Of (H/O) Vaccination**
   (Ensure complete vaccination history)

(2) **Onset :**
   Congenital ; since birth, Neonate, Infancy,
   Adolescence, Age Group;Decade.
   Manifestation: Noticed lesion since when,

(3) **If Congenital Lesion** became symptomatic since when.
   H/O other Associated Cong. Anomalies
   H/O Prenatal & Ante Natal Problems :
   During Pregnancy : H/O Infectious Dis. Contact, ? Treatment.

(4) **H/O Delivery**: ? Obstructed Labour, Difficult Delivery, Home
               Any other Medication (? Trimester, ? Medicine)

   Dai Conducted, Institutional: Normal Delivery full term/pre term,

   Irradiation (X Rays etc)
   H/O Episiotomy, Forceps Application, LSCS
   Etc

(5) **Other Children Overall Health**: ? Problems ? Treatment

(6) **Overall Health of Parents** : ? Problems ? Treatment

   Otherwise Obstetrical history of Mother
   Family H/O Disease: Maternal/Paternal Generations etc.

(7) **Above Mentioned being must ensured Salient Features beside,**
   Routine Cl. Approach to a Paediatric pt.
   (Cl. History, Cl. Exam., Management Etc.)

'FEMALE SURGICAL PATIENTS'

Beside Routine Clinical History Taking, Exams. Etc.
For Systemic Dis. Lesion,
Followings Are Necessory Details In Female Surgical Patients:

Social History: Significant Social History, If Any

Menstrual History: **Menarchae**: Age Of Onset Of Mensuration

    Meno pause: Age of Mensuration cessation

Discharge P/V: Colour, Smell, Amount, Time, Duration,Increased Flow/ Association With Pain Etc.

Menstruation: Regular / Irregular/Cycle

Dysfunctional Uterine Bleeding (D.U.B) Etc.

Obstetrical History: **No. of Children, Age of Last Child Birth**,

    Significant Details of Deliveries;

    H/O LSCS, Abortions Etc.

- History To Confirm Gestation By LMP (Last Menstrual Period), Urine Preganancy Test & Or USG; For Choice of Safe Medication.

- H/O **Breast Feeding**; ? Adv. For Restriction/Cessation,   ? Medicines Regulation

Yes/No, Method Adopted:Barrier Contraception,Condom,

Contraception: Oral Contraceptive Etc

Tubectomy/
Vasectomy Details Etc.

CLINICAL PATHOLOGY DATA

Blood Examination

(1) Blood Urea :
Normal 20-40 mgm/10 c.c.
Raised in Primary rental disease
Lower urinary tract obstruction
Dehydration
Intestinal Obstruction
Diarrhoea

(2) Serum creatinine :
Normal 0.9 to 1.5 mg%

(3) Blood non protein nitrogen
Normal 20-40 mgm/100 c.c.
Raised in (as blood urea)

(4) Bleeding time :
Normal 2-6 minutes
Raised in Thrombocytopaenia
Leukaemia
Normal in Haemophelia

(5) Clotting time :
Normal 5-10 minutes
Raised in Haemophelia
obstructive Jaundice
Normal in Purpura

(6) Prothrombin Time :
Normal 12, 16 seconds
Raised Liver diseases
Obstructive Jaundice

(7) Platelet count :
Normal 270,000-660,000 cmm.
Lowered in Hypersplenism
Purpura haemorrhagica,
Acute leukaemia
Excessive Radium and
deep-ray therapy

(8) Sedimentation Rate :
Normal less than 10 mm/1 hour
Raised in Tuberculosis
Many general diseases

(9) Blood Cholesterol :
Normal 120-220 mgm/100 c.c.
Raised in Obstructive Jaundice
Hypothyroidism
Nephrosis
Diabetes mellitus
Pregnancy
Lowerd in-Hyperthyroidism

(10) Blood sugar (Fasting) :
Normal 80-120 mgm/100 c.c.
Raised in diabetes mellitus
Hyperpituitarism
Hyperthyroidism
Some Cerebral lesions

(11) Blood Proteins :
Normal 6-1 gm/100 c.c.
Lowerd in Chronic Liver disease
Malnutrition
Nephriti
After burns

(12) Albumin :
Normal 4.4-5.3 gm/100 c.c

(13) A.G. Ratio .
Normal A. G. Ratio 1.7/1
Lowered in liver diseases

(14) Cephalin Cholesterol Test :
Normal Negative
Positive in liver damage

(15) Colloidal gold Test same as (13)

(16) Thymol Turbidity Test :
Normal Less than 4 units
Raised in Liver damage

(17) Alkaline Phospatese :
Normal 5.10 King Armstrong unit
1.5-4 Bodansky units
Raised in Obstructive Jaundice
Hyperparathyroidism
secondary Carcinomatosis bone
Lowered in scurvy

(18) Bilirubin :
Normal 0.1.-0.5 mgm/100 c.c.
Raised in Obstructive Jaundice
Acute massive necrosis Liver
Infective hapatitis

(19) Ven den Borgh reaction :
Direct positive in as (17)
Delayed Direct positive in Haemolytic
Jaundice,Toxic Jaundice
Indirect positive in Acholuric Jaundice

(20) Calcium :
Normal 9-11 mgm.
Raised in Hyperparathyroidism
Hypervitaminosis D
Multiple myelomatosis
Prolonged immobilization
Lowered in Hypoparathyroidism
Uraemia
Rickets

(21) Acid phosphatase :
1.2-3.1 KingArmstrongs Units
Raised In Ca Ptostate

Serum Amylase, Serum Lipase, Peritoneal Fluid Amylase

Students Are Advised Accuaintance With Recently Available, Latest Bio-Chemical, Microbiology, Pathology Tests, Esp. Serology, Immunology: Elisa,Polymerase Chain Reaction (PCR), Immunoglobulin Studies,Tumor Markers Etc. For Various Diseases, As Encountered In Day To Day Practice.

Normal Values Of Common Laboratory Tests :

Hematologic	Men	Women
Hemoglobin	13.5–18 g/dL	12–16 g/dL
Hematocrit	40–54%	38–47%
Red blood cells (RBC)	4.6–6.2 million/mm3	4.2–5.4 million/mm3
Mean corpuscular volume (MCV)	76–100 (micrometer)3	76–100 (micrometer)3
Mean corpuscular hemoglobin (MCH)	27–33 picogram	27–33 picogram
Mean corpuscular hemoglobin concentration (MCHC)	33–37 g/dL	33–37 g/dL
Erythrocyte sedimentation rate (ESR)	C20 mm/hr	C30 mm/hr
Leukocytes (WBC)	5000–10,000/mm3	5000–10,000/mm3
Neutrophils	54–75% (3000–7500/mm3)	54–75% (3000–7500/mm3)
Bands	3–8% (150–700/mm3)	3–8% (150–700/mm3)
Eosinophils	1–4% (50–400/mm3)	1–4% (50–400/mm3)
Basophils	0–1% (25–100/mm3)	0–1% (25–100/mm3)
Monocytes	2–8% (100–500/mm3)	2–8% (100–500/mm3)
Lymphocytes	25–40% (1500–4500/mm3)	25–40% (1500–4500/mm3)
T lymphocytes	60–80% of lymphocytes	60–80% of lymphocytes
B lymphocytes	10–20% of lymphocytes	10–20% of lymphocytes
Platelets	150,000–450,000/mm3	150,000–450,000/mm3
Prothrombin time (PT)	9.6–11.8 sec	9.5–11.3 sec
Partial thromboplastin time (PTT)	30–45 sec	30–45 sec
Bleeding time (duke)	1–3 min	1–3 min
Bleeding Time (ivy)	3–6 min	3–6 min
(template)	3–6 min	3–6 min

INVESTIGATION	RESULT	NORMAL RANGE
DIABETIC PROFILE		
Blood Glucose (Fasting)		70-110mg/dl
Blood Glucose (Post parendial)		70-120mg/dl
Blood Glucose (Random)		<140mg/dl
Haemoglobin A1C (Hb A1C)		4.5-7% of total Diabetic with metabolic Imbalance>8.5
RENAL FUNCTION PROFILE		
Blood Urea		15-40mg/dl
Serum Creatinine		Male: 0.5-1.2mg/dl Female: 0.6-0.9mg/dl
Blood Urea Nitrogen		82mg/dl
Serum Osmolality		275-295 mOsmol/kg
Serum Uric Acid		Male: 3.1-7.0mg/dl Female: 2.5-5.6mg/dl
ARTERIAL BLOOD ANALYSIS		
pH		7.39-7.45
pCO_2		32-45mmhg
Bicarbonate		24-30 mmol/L
LIPID PROFILE		
Serum Cholesterol (Total)		140-250mg/dl
Serum Triglyceride		Male 40-160mg/dl Female 35-135mg/dl
Serum HDL		(mg/dl) male female Prognostically> 55>65 Fabourable Standard risk level 35-35 45-65 Risk Indicator <35 <45
Serum LDL		(mg/dl) male Female Reduced risk for CHD <50 <63 Increadses rick > 172 > 167 For CHD
Serum VLDL		Upto 45 mg/dl

HORMONAL INVESTIGATIONS

INVESTIGATION	RESULT	NORMAL RANGE
THYROID PROFILE		
Serum T3 (Free)		1.4-4.2 pgm/ml
Serum T4 (Free)		0.8-2.0 ngm/ml
Serum TSH (Total)		0.3-6.2mlU/ml
Thyroxine-binding globulin:12 – 30 Mgm/L (TBG) Thyroglobulin (TG):1.5-30 pmol/L Or 1-30µg/ml Parathyroid hormone (PTH):10-17- To 65-70 pg/ml Or 1.1-1.8 To 6.9-7.5pmol/L Calcitonin:5ngm/L Or 15 pgm/L (Cutoff against medullary thyroid cancer)		
INFERTILITY PROFILE: L.H.		Female (Mensurating) Folicular Phase – 0.8-10.5IU/L Ovulatory Phase 18.4-61.2U/L Luteal Phase 0.8-10.5IU/L Post Menopause 8.2-40IU/L Male 0.78-7.4IU/L
FSH		Female (Mensurating) Folicular Phase-3-12mlU/L OVulatory Phase 18-22mlU/L Luteal Phase 2-12mlU/L Post Menopause 35-151mlU/L Male 1-14mlU/L
Prolactin		Adult Women Non Pregnant 1.2-15ng/ml Menopause 1.1-12ng/ml Adult Man 1.5-12ng/ml
Testosterone		Adult women<0.6ng/ml Post menopause<0.8ng/ml Boys before puberty 0.31-2ng/ml Adult men 3.5-8.G ng/ml
B-HCG		Time after conception (IU/L) 1st Week 10-30 2nd Week 30-100 3rd Week 100-1000 4th Week 1000-10000 2nd3rd month 30000-100000 2nd trimester 10000-30000 3rd trimester 5000-15000
Progesterone		Adult Women Folicular Phase 0.2-1.4ng/ml Luteal Phase 4-25ng.ml Menopause 0.1-1ng/ml Normal Men 0.1-1ng/ml
OTHER HORMONE		
S. CORTISOL		8Am-12PM-50-250ng/ml 12PM-8PM-50-150ng/ml 8PM-8PM-0-100ng/ml Children 16-18 yers 24-290ng/ml

TUMOUR MARKERS

Investigations	RESULT	NORMAL RANGE
CA-125		0-35U/ml
CEA		Non Smoker<5 ng/ml Smoker<10ng/ml
PSA		<40 years 0.2.0 ng/ml >40 years 0.4.0 ng/ml
AFP		Normal healthy<8.5ng/ml High risk patient suggesting hepatocellular carcinorma-100-350ng/ml Indication of hepatocellular carcinoma>350ng/ml

IMMUNOLOGY
ACUTE PHASE PROTEINS
MARKERS OF INFLAMMATION.

Test	Patient	Lower limit	Upper limit	Unit	Com-mnts
Erythrocyte sedimentation rate (ESR)	Male	0	Age÷2	mm/hr	ESR increase with age and tends to be higher in female
	Female		(Age+10)÷2		
C-reactive protein (CRP)	n/a		5/ 6	mg/L	
			200/240	nmol/L	
Alpha 1-antitrypsin (AAT)		20/22	38/ 53	µmol/L	
		89/97	170/230	mg/dL	

ISOTYPES OF ANTIBODIES
FURTHER INFORMATION: *ANTIBODY*

Test	Patient	Lower limit	Upper limit	Unit	Comments
IgA		70/110	360 /560		
IgD		0.5	3.0		
IgE	Adult	0.01	0.04	mg/dL	
IgG		800	1800		
IgM		54	220		

ORAL GTT		
	Plasma Glucose (PG) Leve(mg/dl)	Reducing Substances in Urine
Fasting		
First Hour		
Second Hour		
Normal glucose tolerance-2 hour PG>=140mg/dl&<200mg/dl Provisional diabetic diagnosis-2hour PG>200mg/dl		

BODY FLUID ANALYSIS	
ADA	10-25 U/L Suspected 30-40 U/L Storng Sustpectedc>40-60 U/L Positive > 60 U/L For CSF Positive> 10 U/L

CEREBROSPINAL FLUID

Cell count	$<4 \times 10^6/L$
Glucose	2-4mmol/L
Proteins (total)	0.20-0.45 g/L

Reference Ranges For Other Molecules In CSF

Substance	Lower Limit	Upper Limit	Unit	Corresponds To % Of That In Plasma
Glucose	50	80[13]	Mg/Dl	~60%
	2.2/ 2.8	3.9/ 4.4]	Mmol/L	
Protein	15	40 / 45	Mg/Dl	~1%
Albumin	7.8	40	Mg/Dl	0 - 0.7% - Corresponding To An *Albumin (Csf/Serum) Quotient* Of 0 To 7 $X10^{-3}$

CEREBROSPINAL FLUID

Cause	Appearance	Polymorphonuclear Leukocytes	Lympho Cytes	Protein	Glucose
Pyogenic Bacterial Meningitis	Yellowish, Turbid	Markedly Increased	Slight Increaseor Normal	Markedly Increased	Decrease
Viral Meningitis	Clear Fluid	Slightly Increased Or Normal	Marked Increase	Slightly Increased Or Normal	Normal
Tuberculous Meningitis	Yellowish And Viscous	Slightly Increased Or Normal	Marked Increase	Increased	Decrease
Fungal Meningitis	Yellowish And Viscous	Slightly Increased Or Normal	Marked Increase	Slight Increase Or Normal	Normal Or Decrease

URINE EXAMINATION

Test		Lower limit	Upper limit	Unit	Comments
Urine Specific Gravity		1.003	1.030	no unit	This Test Detects The Ion Concentration Of Urine. Small Amounts Of Protein Or Ketoacidosis Tend To Elevate The Urine's Specific Gravity(SG). This Value Is Measured Using A Urinometer And Indicates Whether You Are Hydrated Or Dehydrated. If The SG Of Your Urine Is Under 1.010 You Are Hydrated. If Your Urine SG Is Above 1.020, You Are Dehydrated.
Osmolality		400	n/a	mOsm/kg	
pH		5	7	(unitless)	
Bacterial cultures	By Urination	–	100,000	Colony Forming Units Per Millilitre (CFU/Ml)	Bacteriuria Can Be Confirmed If A Single Bacterial Species Is Isolated In A Concentration Greater Than 100,000 Colony Forming Unitsper Millilitre Of Urine In Clean-Catch Midstream Urine Specimens (One For Men, Two Consecutive Specimens With The Same Bacterium For Women).*Further Information: Bacteriuria*
	By Bladder Catheterisation	–	100		For Urine Collected Via Bladder Catheterisation, The Threshold Is 100 Colony Forming Units Of A Single Species Per Millilitre. *Further Information: Bacteriuria*

- **Haematuria-Associated With** Kidney Stones, Infections, Tumors **And Other Conditions**
- Pyuria – **Associated With** Urinary Infections
- Eosinophiluria – **Associated With** Allergic Interstitial Nephritis, Atheroembolic Disease
- Red Blood Cell Casts – **Associated With** Glomerulonephritis, Vasculitis, Malignant Hypertension
- White Blood Cell Casts – **Associated With** Acute Interstitial Nephritis, **Exudative** Glomerulonephritis, **Severe** Pyelonephritis
- **(Heme) Granular Casts – Associated With** Acute Tubular Necrosis
- Crystalluria – **Associated With** Acute Urate Nephropathy **(Or "Acute Uric Acid Nephropathy", AUAN)**
- Calcium Oxalatin – **Associated With** Ethylene Glycol **Toxicity**
- **Urine Sugar Levels KetonUria: Diabetic Conditions**
- **Bile Salts, Bile Pigments Etc: Jaundice Patients**
- Drug Test Pregnancy Test, **Measures** HCG **Levels In Urine**

URINE ANALYSIS	
24 Hr Urine Protein	21-120 mg/day
24 Hr Urine Creatinine	1000-1500 mg/day
Creatinine dearance test	Men 95-156 ml/Min Women 95-160 ml/min
Spot Urine	
Micro albumin	0-35 mg/day

URINE ANALYSIS

Calcium	<7.3 mmol/day
Chloride	110-250 mmol/day
Creatinine	6.2-17.7 mmol/day
Osmolality	100-1200 mOsm/kg
Potassium	25-120 mmol/day
Protein	<0.15 g/day
Sodium	

HUMAN FAECES

Meconium (Sometimes Erroneously Spelled *Merconium*) Is A Newborn Baby's First Feces.

Bristol Stool Chart
Bristol Stool Scale

The Bristol Stool Chart Or Bristol Stool Scale Is A Medical Aid Designed To Classify The Form Of Human Feces Into Seven Categories. Sometimes Referred To In The Uk As The "Meyers Scale
The Seven Types Of Stool Are:

1. Separate Hard Lumps, Like Nuts (Hard To Pass)
2. Sausage-Shaped But Lumpy
3. Like A Sausage But With Cracks On The Surface
4. Like A Sausage Or Snake, Smooth And Soft
5. Soft Blobs With Clear-Cut Edges
6. Fluffy Pieces With Ragged Edges, A Mushy Stool
7. Watery, No Solid Pieces. Entirely Liquid

Types 1 And 2 Indicate Constipation. Types 3 And 4 Are Optimal, Especially The Latter, As These Are The Easiest To Pass. Types 5–7 Are Associated With Increasing Tendency To Diarrhea Or Urgency.

FECAL CONTAMINATION

The main pathogens that are commonly looked for in feces include:

- *Bacteroides* species
- *Salmonella* and *Shigella*
- *Yersinia* tends to be incubated at 30 °C (86 °F), which is cooler than usual
- *Campylobacter* incubated at 42 °C (108 °F), in a special environment
- *Aeromonas*
- *Candida* if the person is immunosuppressed (e.g., undergoing cancer treatment)
- *E. coli* O157 if blood is visible in the stool sample
- *Cryptosporidium*

- *Entamoeba histolytica*

UNDIGESTED FOOD REMNANTS

FAECAL MARKERS

Various Markers That Are Indicative Of Various Diseases And Conditions Eg

- Fecal Calprotectin **Levels Indicate An Inflammatory Process Such As** Crohn's Disease, Ulcerative -Colitis

  And Neoplasms (Cancer).

- **Faecal Lactoferrin**

<u>FECES ANALYSIS FOR:</u> **Any** Fecal Occult Blood**, Indicative Of** Gastrointestinal Bleeding**.**

INVESTIGATION	RESULT	NORMALRANGE
DIABETIC PROFILE		
Blood Glucose(Fasting)		70-110mg/dl
Blood Glucose (Post parendial)		90-130mg/dl
Blood Glucose(Random)		<140mg/dl
Haemoglobin A1C (Hb A1C)		4.5-7% of total Diabetic with metabolic imbalance>8.5
RENAL FUNCTION PROFILE		
Blood Urea		15-40mg/d
Serum Creatinine		Male: 0.5-1.2mg/dl Female: 0.6-0.9mg/d
Blood Urea Nitrogen		8-20mg/dl
Serum Osmolality		285-295 mOsmol/kg serum water
Serum Uric Acid		Male: 3.1-7.0mg/dl Female: 2.6-5.6mg/dl
ARTERIAL BLOOD ANALYSIS		
pH		7.39-7.45
pCO_2		32-45mmHg
pO_2		72-104mmHg
Bicarbonate		24-30 mmol/L
LIPID PROFILE		
Serum Cholesterol (Total)		140-250mg/dl
Serum Triglyceride		Male 40-160mg/dl Female 35-135mg/dl
Serum HDL		(mg/dl) male female Prognostically >55 >65 favourable Standard risk level 35-55 45-65 Risk Indicator <35 <45
Serum LDL		(mg/dl) male female Reduced risk for CHD <50 <62 Increased risk >172 >197 for CHD
Serum VLDL		Upto 45 mg/dl
Lipid Ratio		
PANCREATIC PROFILE		
Serum Amylase (37°c)		35-180U/L
Serum Lipase (37°c)		Upto 60U/L

INVESTIGATION	RESULT	NORMALRANGE
LIVER FUNCTION PROFILE		
Serum Bilirubin (Total)		At Birth upto 5mg/dl 5days up to 12 mg/dl 1 month upto 15mg/dl Adults up to 1.1mg/dl
Serum Bilirubin- Direct (Conjugated)		Adults upto 0.3 mg/dl
Serum Bilirubin-Indirect (uncojugated)		0.1-0.8 mg/dl
Serum Protein (Total)		Normal born babies 4.0-7gm/d Children from 3 year and Adults 6.6-8.7gm/dl
Serum Albumin		3.5-5.5 gm/dl
Serum Globulin		2.0-3.5 gm/dl
A:G (RATIO)		0.9-2.3
SGPT (ALT) (37°c)		5-40 IU/L
SGOT (AST)(37°c)		5-45 IU/L
Serum Alkaline Phosphatase (ALP) (37°c)		Male20-50yrs 40-88 U/L >60yrs 43-88 U/L Female20-50yrs 28-98U/L >60yrs 40-111U/l
Gama Glutamyl transferase (GGT) (37°c)		Male 10-45 U/L Female 5-32 U/L
CARDIAC PROFILE		
CPK-NAC (37°C)		Male 20-190 U/L Female 20-170 U/L
CPK-MB (37°c)		0-25 U/L
Troponin I/Troponin T (Card test)		
Hs-CRP		Upto 6mg/dl
LDH (Total)		240-480 U/L
INORGANIC SUBSTANCES		
Serum Calcium (Total)		8.5-10.5 mg/dl
Serum Phosphorus (Total)		Male 2.1-4.5mg/dl Female 1.6-6.8mg/dl
Serum Sodium (Ionized)		135-155 mmol/L
Serum Potassium (Ionized)		3.5-5.5 mmol/L
Serum Chloride (Ionized)		95-110 mmol/L
Serum Lithium (Ionized)		Up to 0.003 mmol/l
Other Investigation (if any)		

HORMONAL INVESTIGATION

INVESTIGATION	RESULT	NORMALRANGE
THYROID PROFILE		
Serum T3 (Free)		1.4-4.2 pgm/ml
Serum T4 (Free)		0.8-2.0 ngm/ml
Serum TSH (Total)		0.3-6.2mIU/ml
INFERTILITY PROFILE		
LH		Female (Mensurating) Folicular Phase-0.8-10.5IU/L Ovulatory Phase 18.4-61.2IU/L Lutea Phase 0.8-10.5IU/L Post Menopause 8.2-40IU/L Male 0.7-7.4IU/L
FSH		Female (Mensurating) Folicular Phase 3-12mIU/L Ovulatory Phase 8-22mIU/L Luteal Phase 2-12 mIU/L Post Menopause 35 151mIU/L Male 1-14mIU/L
Prolactin		Adult Women Non Pregnant 1.2-20ng/ml Post Menopause 1.5 -19ng/ml Adult Man 1.5-12ng/ml
Testosterone		Adult women<0.6ng/ml Post menopause<0.8ng/ml Boys before puberty 0.31-2ng/ml Adult men 3.5-8.6ng/ml
ß-HCG		Time after conception (IU/L) 1st week 10-30 2nd week 30-100 3rd week 100-1000 4th week 1000-10000 2nd-3rd month 30000-100000 2nd trimester 10000-30000 3rd trimester 5000-15000
Progesterone		Adult Women Folicular Phase 0.2-1.4ng/ml Luteal Phase 4-25ng.ml Menopause 0.1-1ng/ml Normal Men 0.1-1ng/ml
OTHER HORMONE		
Cortisol		8AM-12PM-50-250ng/ml 12PM-8PM-50-150ng/ml 8PM-8PM-0-100ng/ml Children 16-18 yers 24-290ng/ml

*References for normal-HARISON & WHO Norms

TUMOUR MARKERS

INVESTIGATION	RESULT	NORMALRANGE
CA-125		0-35U/ml
CEA		Non Smoker<5 ng/ml Smoker<10ng/ml
PSA		<40 year 0-2.0ng/ml >40 years 0-4.0ng/ml
AFP		Normal healthy<8.5ng/ml High risk patient suggesting hepatocellular carcinoma-100-350ng/ml Indication of hepatocellular carcinoma>350ng/ml

ORAL GTT

	Plasma Glucose (PG) Level(mg/dl)	Reducing substances in urine
Fasting		
First Hour		
Second Hour		

Normal glucose tolerance-2 hour PG<140mg/dl
Impaired glucose tolerance-2 hour PG>=140mg/dl&<200mg/dl
Provisional diabetic diagnosis-2 hour PG>200mg/dl

BODY FLUID ANALYSIS

ADA		10-25 U/L Suspected 30-40 U/L Strong Suspected>40-60 U/L Positive>60 U/L For CSF Postivie>10U/L
CSF (Micro Protein)		20-50 mg/dl
CSF (Glucose)		40-70mg/dl
Other Body Fluid		
Total Protein		
Glucose		

URINE ANALYSIS

24 Hr Urine Protein		21-120mg/day
24 Hr Urine Creatinine		1000-1500mg/day
Creatinine clearance test		Men95-156ml/min Women 95-160ml/min
Micro albumin		0-35 mg/day
Spot Urine		

SECTION:(A)
HISTORY SHEETS

Should Include Following Type Of Cases, Necessarily In,
➤ **Allotted Patients Record Maintainence,**

- Head Injuries Brain tumors, Other Neurological Lesions
- Thyroid Swellings, Other Neck Swellings.

  - Head & Neck Tumors, Swellings, Salivary Glands, Oral Cavity Lesions.
  - Breast Lumps, Pathologies
  - Oesophagus, Gastric & Duodenal Diseases
  - Pancreatitis, Biliary, Intestinal Colics, Appendicular Pathologies

- Gall Bladder Diseases : Stone Dis., Malignancy Etc., Hepato-Biliary Dis., Obstructive Jaundice,

- Ano - Rectal Cases, Pilonidal Disease.

  - Genito-Urinary case : Stone Disease, Infections, Haematuria, Malignancy, Prostatism.

    - Inguino-Scrotal Swellings

    - Ext. Genitalia Lesions

    - Peripheral Vascular Diseases, Progressive Necrotizingic Fascitis; Cellulitis

- Skin & Soft Tissue Swellings of different Size, shape, Site & Tissue Involvements.

  - Abdominal Lumps of different organ of orgin.

    Operative & Non Op. Surgical Problems
    - Abdominal Emergencies with or without Associated Affections, Trauma,

    - Chest –Cases : Trauma, Tumor, Chr. Disease manifestations
  - Fractures (Complete Medico legal Aspects of every Case)

  - Diseases of Bones

  - Diseases of Joints

  - Paediatric Surgical Cases.

'HISTORY SHEETS'
Long Cases & Short Cases,
At Least (4) Short Cases, Necessary.

Case No.	Name of Patients	Ward/Bed	Diagnosis	Surgeon I/C
1.				
2.				
3.				
4.				
5.				
6.				
7.				
8.				
9.				
10.				
11.				
12.				
13.				
14.				
15.				

Include (1) Case Each From Special Surgical Wards:
Surgical ICU (SICU) & Burn Ward.

CASE NO ....WD.................BED NO..............SURGEON ....

Occupation

Patient's Name

Marital Status

Age

Permanent Home Address

Sex

Date of Admission

Date of discharge

Diagnosis.

CLINICAL HISTORY

CHIEF COMPLAINTS : 1.

2.

3.

HISTORY OF PRESENT ILLNESS :
(The Sequence Of Events Must Be Clearly Brought Out)

PREVIOUS ILLNESS (If Any):

HABITS : Secondary/Active/Hard labour

Tobacco/Alcohol/other intoxicants

FAMILY HISTORY : Age if alive   If dead, age at death & its cause

Father

Mother

Brother

Sister

Wife/Husband

SOCIAL STATUS : Family Income

PHYSICAL EXAMINATION

GENERAL EXAMINATION

Appearance :

Build :

Nutritional State :

Hydration :

Anaemia :

Obvious Focal Sepsis, Teeth & Gums

    Tonsils

    Ear
    Skin

Pulse :

B. P.

Respiration

Temperature

Cyanosis

Clubbing

Jaundice

Oedema

Lympth-Adenopathy

Others--------

CERVICAL LYMPTH NODES LEVELS
Level Ia-SubMental Δ Nodes
Level Ib - SubMandibular Δ Nodes
Level II- Upper Deep Cervical Nodes
Level III- Middle Deep Cervical Nodes
Level IV- Lower Deep Cervical Nodes
Level V- Post. Δ L. Nodes
Level VI- Ant. Cervical L. Nodes
Level VII- Upper Mediastinal L.Nodes

SYSTEMIC EXAMINATION :

Cardio respiratory Reserve :   Breath Holding Time :

                                          Exercise Tolerance :

   Heart :   Peripheral Blood Vessels :

Lungs :

Nervous System :

DIETETIC HABITS : (Average Daily Calorie Intake Etc.)

"SKETCH DIAGRAMS EXAMPLES:PHYSICAL SIGNS RECORDS"

LOCAL EXAMINATION (RULE OF NINE Etc.)

FRONT **BACK**

CHEST, ABDOMEN, INGUINAL
REGION, EXT. GENITALIA Etc.

HEAD & NECK

CARCINOMATOUS

RODENT

SEPTIC

TUBERCULAR

SYPHILITIC

ULCERS

THORAX (LUNGS, MEDIASTINUM ETC.)

B / L BREAST

PER RECTAL EXAM. (PERI-ANAL REGION,
PROSTATE AND VESICLES ETC.)

SUPERIOR, INFERIOR
EXTREMITIES Etc.

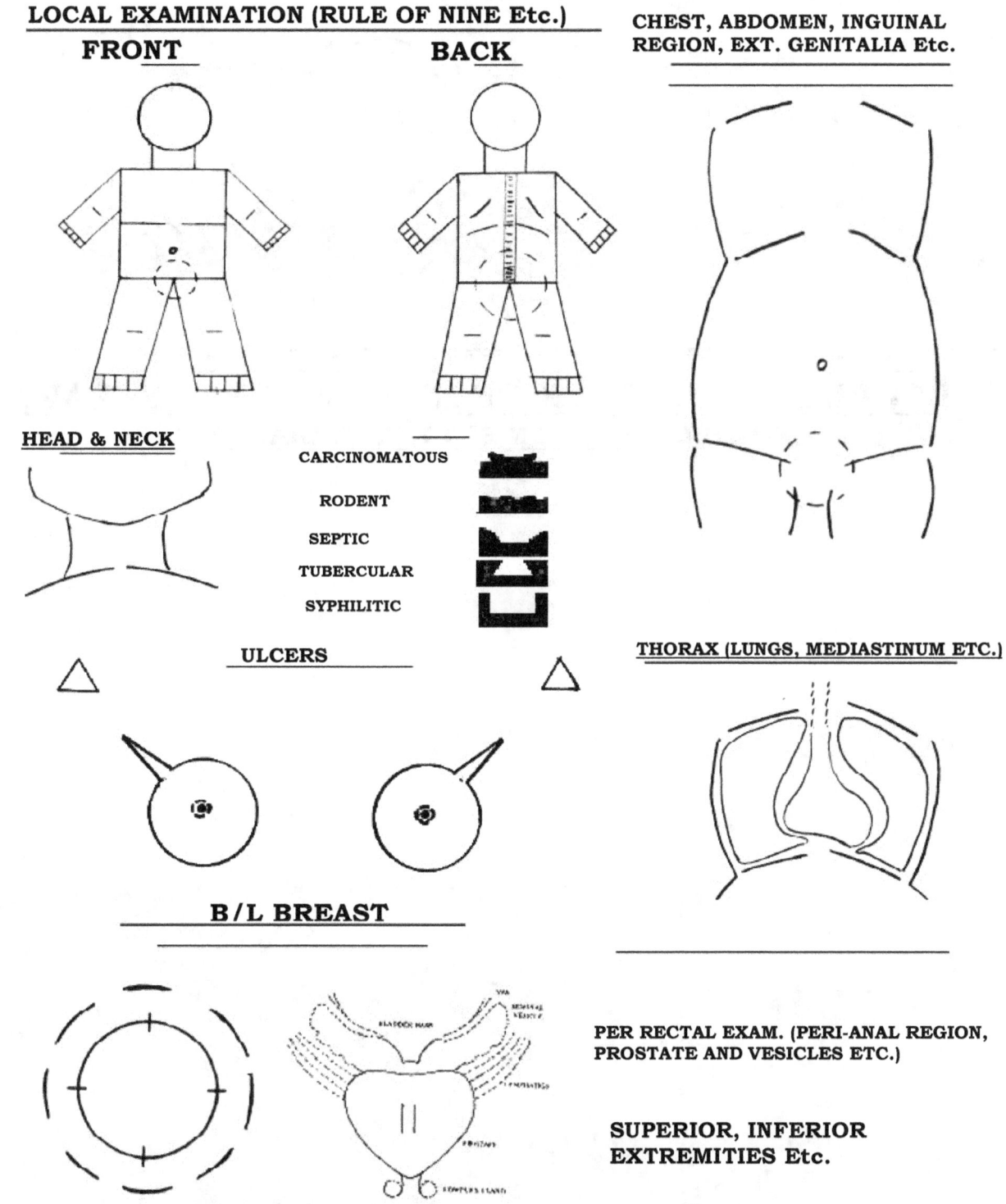

Alimentary System : (including Rectal Examination)

UPPER G.I.T	LOWER G.I.T	URINARY SYSTEM
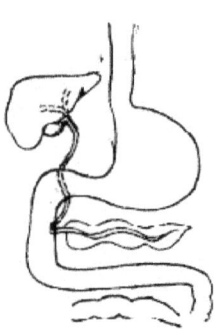	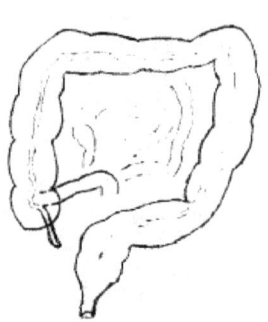	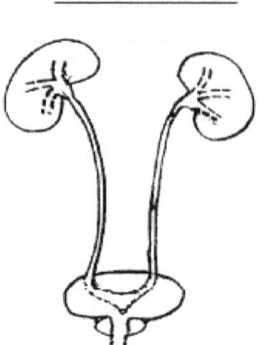

==

LOCAL EXAMINATION OF INVOLVED BODY- PARTS
(FOR ILLUSTRATION BY SKETCH DIAGRAMS)

'CLINICAL IMPRESSION'

Provisional Diagnosis :
 Points in favour :1.
                    2.
                    3.
                    4.

Differential Diagnosis :
                    1.
                    2.
                    3.
                    4.

Investigations Suggested And Findings
Expected :   1.
                    2.
                    3.
                    4.
                    5.

Points Against :
1.
2.
3.
4.

Reports of Investigation :

Investigations	Date		
Blood: Hb% DLC ESR TLC			
Urine: Alb. Sugar Bile Microscopic			
Blood Sugar: Post-Prandial Fastings Others			

Radiological Investigations :

PROGRESS REPORT

SPECIAL PREOPERATIVE PREPARATION :

PREMEDICATION   1.

(Dose & Time)   2.

                             3.

                             4.

ANAESTHESIA USED: 1.

                             2.

                             3.

                             4.

OPERATIVE STEPS :

    Position of the Patient:

    Incision & Exposure :

    Findings :

    OPERATION NOTES
Operative Procedure Performed (Described In Detail)

Any Special Remarks :
(Including Comment Upon Histopathology Specimen, Post-operative Period,
Recovery,Complications Etc, With Condition at Discharge, Medico-Legal Records Etc.)

(To Be Filled Every Day In Serious Cases And During 10 Post- Operative Days, AndEvery Third Day In Others. Mention Observations Pertaining To A Case Any Special Investigations Done And Daily Treatment Administered.)

Dated   **Condition Of Patient**   **Treatment Given**

FINAL APPRAISAL: (Write Your Overall Impression Of Case At The Time Of Disharge Or When You Leave The Case. The Histopathological Diagnosis. If Any And The Result Of Treatment Sould Be Indicated.)

Signature of Surgeon

Signature of Student

SECTION:B "SURGICAL PATHOLOGY"

☐ **AMONGST FOLLOWING COMMON SURGICAL SPECIMENS:**

☐ Excisional Biopsy Sp. of various body swellings, Lipoma, Fibroma, Neuroma, Cystic Swellings, Lympth Adenopathy, Lymphoma, Caseated Lymph nodes Specimens Etc.

☐ Head & Neck Tumors : Tongue, Lip, Cheek, Salivary Glands Etc.

☐ Thyroidectomy Specimens: Muitinodular Goitre, Solitary Cyst, Carcinoma Etc. Other Neck Swellings Specimens.
Chest Tumors Specimens Etc.

☐ Fibroadenoma, Fibroadenosis, Fibrocystic Dis., Carcinoma Breast, Gynaecomezia Etc.Mastectomy Specimens.

☐ Carcinoma Esophagus, Stricture oesophagus, DU Perforation, Stomach Growths

Liver Cirrhosis, Hepatoma, Hydatid Cyst of Liver, Splenectomy Specimens

Gall Bladder Diseases : Chronic Cholecystitis,Cholelithiasis, Ca G.B,

Acute Appendicitis, Mucocele of Appendix, Maeckel's Diverticulum, Diverticular Dis.
Intestinal Obstruction due to round worms Etc., Intussusception, Volvulus,Typhoid Ulcers of ileum Amoebic Ulcers, Bacillary dysentery Etc.Carcinoma Colon, Carcinoma Rectum Etc.

☐ Ano-Rectal Pathology Specimens

Renal Cell Carcinoma,Wilm's tumor Polycystic Kidneys, Hydronephrosis, Nephrectomy, Orchidectomy, Amputation Penis Specimens.
Enlarged Prostate With Secondary Changes In Bladder, Urinary Bladder Tumors,Vesical Calculus

Madura Foot, Jaipur foot
Soft tissue Swellings. Muscle Tumors Etc.

T.B Spine, Osteomyelitis, Oseteo sarcoma, Other Bone Tumors Sp.

& Other Specimens of Academic Interest.

'SURGICAL PATHOLOGY'

S.No.	Specimen/Chart Name	Surgeon I/C
1.		
2.		
3.		
4.		
5.		
6.		
7.		
8.		
9.		
10.		

ASSESMENT REMARKS:

DATE:

TEACHER'S SIGNATURE

SURGICAL PATHOLOGY (1)

SURGICAL PATHOLOGY (2)

SECTION(C):
'SURGICAL RADIO-DIAGNOSIS'

AMONGST FOLLOWINGS X-RAYS :
(PLAIN X-RAY & CONTRAST RADIOLOGY, RADIO-DIAGNOSTICS ETC.)

- ☐ # Of Long Bone, Osteomyetitis, Osteosarcoma, & Others Bone Tumors, Spine #, T B Spine

- ☐ X Ray Chest (PA, AP, Lateral, oblique, Sternal Views) :
  Pulm- Koch's (Variable Disease Stages), Emphysema. Hydropneumothorax, Haemothorax,Haemopneumothorax, Pneumothorax, Etc.
  # Ribs, Primary & or Multiple Secondaries In The Lung, Mediastinal Tumors, Lymph Node Masses, Etc.

- ☐ X Ray Abd. (K.U.B, PA, AP, Lateral Views, Standing/Sitting/Erect Including both Domes Diapharam):
  Gas Under Diaphragm. Multiple Fluid Levels Indicating Intestinal Obstruction.
  Volvulus Of Sigmoid Colon, Intussusception

- ☐ Soft Tissue Shadows of different sizes, shapes & Sites, Calcification due to T.B.nodes

  Calcification Due To Pancreaticolithaisis, Cholelithiasis, Choledocho-Lithiasis
  Urolithiasis (kidney, ureter, urinary Bladder Stones).
  Nephro calcinosis.

- ☐ Barium Swallow : Ca Oesophagus, Stricture, Achalasia, Esophageal Varices Etc.

  Barium Meal,Stomach Duodenum Showing Carcinoma Stomach, Multiple Follow Through : Polyposis of Stomach, Pyloric Stenosis, Intestinal Stricture Etc.
  Barium Enema : Carcinoma Colon, Ca Ano-Rectum, Tumors, Strictures Etc.
  Sinography, Fistulography Other Contrast Radio-Diagnosis Films.
  Intra Venous Pyelography (I.V.P), Micturition Cysto-Urethrography (M.C.U), Retro-Grade Urethrography (R.G.U) & Various Other Genito-Urinary-System Radiology Films,Revealing Stones, Cong. Anamolies, Hydrohephrosis, Pelvi-Calyceal System Dilatations,Pelvi-Ureteric Junction (PUJ) Obstruction, Ureteric Stones, Strictures, Urinary Bladder Stones,Tumors, Refluxes, Urethral Strictures Etc.

- ☐ Ultrasonography, CT Scan/Contrast Enhanced CT Scan, MRI, Doppler's Study.
  Other Radio-Diagnostic Depictions Of Various Body Organs (Normal & Or Diseased Viscera).

'SURGICAL RADIO-DIAGNOSIS'

Sr No.	Illustration Name	Surgeon I/C
1.		
2.		
3.		
4.		
5.		
6.		
7.		
8.		
9.		
10.		

DATE: ASSESMENT REMARKS:

TEACHER'S SIGNATURE

SURGICAL RADIO-DIAGNOSIS:(1)

SURGICAL RADIO-DIAGNOSIS:(2)

SECTION:(D)
'SURGICAL INSTRUMENTS'

AMONGST FOLLOWING COMMON SURGICAL INSTRUMENTS, APPLIANCES :

➢ Chaetel's Forceps, Sponge Holder,Gland Holding Forceps, Small/Medium/Large Size,Straight/Curved Artery Forceps(Hemostats); Kocher's Clamp, Allis, Babcock's,Rt. Angle,Chole-Docholithotomy, CystoLithotomy, PyeloLithotomy Forceps, Needle Holders,Scissors;Heavy,Straight,Curved,Dissecting,Mayo's,Suture Cutting Dissecting/Thumb Forceps(Toothed/Non-Toothed), Intestinal Crushing/Non-Crushing Clamps Etc.

• Retractors Of Various Types:Self-Retaining,Cjerney's,Single/Double Hook, Renal Pelvis(Eye-Lid),Morris/Devar's,Thyroid, Thoracotomy Etc. Rib- Raspatory, Periosteum Elevator, Chisel, Osteotome,Giggle's Saw

• Different Type Of Blades, Needles, Suture Materials.

• Ryles Tube, Drains, Sengstaken Blackmore Tubes,Flatus Tube, Different Types Of Enemas Etc,

Indwelling Catheters, Asepto Syringes, Tourniquet Etc, Various drainage Systems Including Suction drainages.

Cystostomy Trocar, Suprapubic Catheter (Supra-cath) etc.

• Intercostal Chest Tube Drainage System (ICD), Aspiration Sets Etc.

Drugs esp. Emergency Tray medications, Anaesthetic agents, Boyle's Apparatus,

Laryngoscope, Endotracheal Intubation Ventilators Etc.

I.V.Fluids Therapy appliances including 3 way connectors, Infusion pumps etc.

• Other Common Use Surgical Appliances Rubber, Sialastic Silicon Tubings,

• C-Arm Image Intensifier, Endoscopy & Laproscopic Instrument Appliance Systems For OrthoPaedic & Surgical Procedures

'SURGICAL INSTRUMENTS'

Sr No.	Instrument/ Appliance Name	Surgeon I/C
1.		
2.		
3		
4.		
5.		
6.		
7.		
8.		
9.		
10.		

DATE: ASSESMENT REMARKS:

TEACHER'S SIGNATURE

SURGICAL INSTRUMENTS:(1)

SURGICAL INSTRUMENTS:(2)

(E) OPD, OT, SPECIAL CASES DUTY DETAILS

Surgical Outpatient Deptt.	From _____ To _____
Subject	Remarks By Teacher
1. Examination of Swelling	
2. " " Ulcer	
3. " " Sinus & Fistula	
4. " " Oral Cavity	
5. " " Thyroid	
6. " " Breast	
7. " " Joint	
8. " " Hernia	
9. " " Abdomen	
10. " Scrotum	
11. " " Rectum	
12. " " Peripheral Nerves	
13. " " Gangrene	
14. " " Urinary System	

UNIT ....   FROM _____ TO _____

Elective Operations

Disease	Oper. Done	Surgeon	Signature
1.			
2.			
3.			
4.			
5.			

Emergency Operations

Disease	Oper. Done	Surgeon	Signature
1.			
2.			
3.			
4.			
5.			

Duty On Special Cases

Name	Diagnosis	No. of Hours Done	Signature
1.			
2.			
3.			
4.			

REMARKS:

'ABOUT THE AUTHOR'

PROF.DR. ANIL K. SAHNI
B.Sc., M.B.B.S., M.S., F.I.C.S., Advanced D.H.A.
SURGEON, UROLOGIST, ENDOSCOPIST, LITHOTRIPSY SPECIALIST.

Address: A-1/F-1 Block-A Dilshad Garden
Delhi-110095 India

Life Member :
Austrian Medical Society
The Association Of Surgeons Of India
Delhi Urological Society
Association Of Minimal Access Surgeons Of India
International Association Of Gastr0-Endosurgeons
Medical Council Of India Reg.No.: **3599(06.01.2005) / 27417(30.05.1983)U.P.**
DATE OF BIRTH : **02-06-1958**

Mobile : **09873083100**
E-Mail : **dranil_sahni@yahoo.co.in**
dranil_sahni@hotmail.com

DR. ANIL K. SAHNI

"QUALIFICATIONS": **PASSED ALL EXAMS IN FIRST ATTEMPT WITH POS**
B.Sc :1977, Rohilkhand University, Bareilly. Merit Position, National Scholarship
M.B.B.S :1983, G.S.V.M. Medical College, Kanpur.
M.S : 1986, G.S.V.M. Medical College, Kanpur.
F.I.C.S :1995-96, International College of Surgeons, Chicago, Illinois, USA.
ADHA (Advanced Diploma Hospital Administration) :
2006, Institute of Health Care Administration,Chennai.
"EXTRA-CURRICULUM":**First Aid Certificate,1968, NSS & NCC Certification,1975-77,**
Joint Treasurer, Physiology Society,1978: Executive Member, Socio-Cultural Society,
G.S.V.M. Medical College, Kanpur, 1982 Etc.,
Sports, Music, Print - Live Media & Others.

"EXPERIENCES"

(A)TEACHING EXPERIENCE:
DEMO./TUTOR/REG./RSO/SR:-GSVM Med.Coll.Kanpur (31.05.83 To 31.08.86);3 Yrs & 3 Months
-MCKR Hosp.& Ayur.Res.Inst.Delhi:(10.11.87 To 30.06.89); 1 Year & 8 Months
-Yashoda Hospital,Ghaziabad..: (1.1.1993 To 1.12.1994); 2 Years
ASSISTANT PROFESSOR (SURGERY) :- SantoshMed.Coll.Ghaziabad:(06.04.98 To 26.03.2001);2 Yrs&11Months
- SRMS IMS,Bareilly:(1.07.2004 To17.05.2006);1Yr & 11 Months
- M.M.C.H., Muzaffarnagar: (18.05.06 To 31.08.07); 1Yr & 4 Months
- M.A.M.C., Agroha (Hisar): (1.09.07 To 31.06.08); 10 Months
ADDITIONAL :Urology,Lithotripsy,Non-Invasive/Minimal Invasive Surgery, Endoscopy,
Surgical Teaching, BPT(Physio-Therapy) Courses, G.J Univ.Hisar.
ASSOCIATE PROFESSOR (SURGERY):-M.A.M.C.,Agroha(Hisar):(1.07.08 To 15.03.09);9Months
-VCSG Govt.Med.Sciences & Res.Inst. Sri-Nagar,Pauri-Garhwal:
{Offi.HOD, Act.MS, As Need},Co-ChairMan'CME','CPD'...,
I/C Med.Edu.Unit; 15/16.03.2009 - Till Date.
PROFESSOR: Forwarded & Recommended w.e.f 01/07/2011,Confirmed MCI.
(B) ASSOCIATED ASSIGNMENTS(TRAINING):**Esteemed Tertiary Care Hospitals, P.G Teaching, DNB Courses:**
-Sir Ganga Ram Hospital, Delhi: (Dec. 1998 To Dec. 2001); About (3) Year
-Narendra Mohan Hospital, Ghaziabad: (08.05.1999 To June 2005); About (6) Years
-Surya Hospital, Delhi:About (4)Years & Others: In Various Capacities , Including "ADMINISTRATION".
(C) FOREIGN ASSIGNMENTS: **-National Iranian Oil Company Hospitals,Iran. - About (1)One Year,**
17.12.1991 To 17.12.1992.
-Aviation & Submarine (Metiga) Hospital, Tripoli, Libya. – About (1) One Year,
26.05.1996 To 25/26. 05. 1997.
Versatile, Wide, Experience in Gen. Surgery, Urology , Lithotripsy & Working Experience Of Other Surgical
Super Specialities, Including Intensive Care (Incharge ICU).
"Advanced Diploma In Health Administration" & • Others : Certification In Process.
*(CME),(CPD),(LLL)...: **Various National & InterNational Medical Education Programmes,Constant Participation**
Throughout, Graduation Onwards, About(>50) . **National & International Conferences, Seminars, Symposiums Etc.**
Participation By Important 'Scientific Studies', Useful Presentations, Discussions,Chairing Session, Publications.
-"3rd AMASI Skill Course", AIIMS, N.Delhi, 29th Nov. - 1st Dec.2006.
-"N.S.V Training Course": PGIMS, Rohtak, March'2008 ; C.S.M Medical University Lucknow, September'2011.
-"Post Graduate Surgical Course", Royal College Of Surgeons Of Edinburgh, U.K, Oct.'2008.
-"MCI Co-Ordinators Orientation Progr.(1Day):MCI BasicWorkshop(3 Days),MCI NodalCentre,CMC,Ludhina:Sept.2009.
-"AIIMS Ultrasound Trauma Lifesupport (AUTLS) Course", ASITECH,ASICON'2010, AIIMS, N.Delhi, 15-20 Dec.2010.
*About (25) : Publications, Including Books; **1."Arabic Language. . ." RNI, I & B Ministry, GOI, 2003, Several Reprints, '**
Supplement',Consideration By UN,ICRC,WHO & Others 2." Students Surgery Manual", Dec.2010. . .
*About (25) : 'Scientific Presentations'; **Computronics Media Publications,Colloborating Trauma,Filariasis,**
Breast Care Global Projects ICMR & Others *About (20): 'Scientific Projects'(In Process): **Common Clinical Entities,**
Useful 'Research Projects' & Or 'Thesis Topics', Including Books; **"Surgery For Physio-Therapists".**
Essentials Of LthoTripsy".
* Name, Selected, Nominated, Proposed, Published with other Esteemed Personalities, of Different Magnitudes,
By Various National & InterNational Reputed Institutions.

"Students' Surgery Manual."
Prof.Dr.Anil K. Sahni

"Students' Surgery Manual."
Prof.Dr.Anil K. Sahni